THE BIBLE CURE® FOR

HIGH CHOLESTEROL

DON COLBERT, M.D.

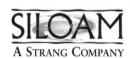

SILOAM
A STRANG COMPANY

Most Strang Communications/Charisma House/Siloam products are available at special quantity discounts for bulk purchase for sales promotions, premiums, fund-raising and educational needs. For details, write Strang Communications/Charisma House/ Siloam, 600 Rinehart Road, Lake Mary, Florida 32746, or telephone (407) 333-0600.

The Bible Cure for High Cholesterol
by Don Colbert, M.D.
Published by Siloam
A Strang Company
600 Rinehart Road
Lake Mary, Florida 32746
www.siloam.com

Unless otherwise noted, all Scripture quotations are from the Holy Bible, New Living Translation, copyright © 1996. Used by permission of Tyndale House Publishers, Inc., Wheaton, IL 60189. All rights reserved.

Scripture quotations marked KJV are from the King James Version of the Bible.

Library of Congress Catalog Card Number:
2003110912

International Standard Book Number:
1-59185-241-2

This book is not intended to provide medical advice or to take the place of medical advice and treatment from your personal physician. Readers are advised to consult their own doctors or other qualified health professionals regarding the treatment of their medical problems. Neither the publisher nor the author takes any responsibility for any possible consequences from any treatment, action or application of medicine, supplement, herb or preparation to any person reading or following the information in this book. If readers are taking prescription medications, they should consult with their physicians and not take themselves off of medicines to start supplementation without the proper supervision of a physician.

05 06 07 08 — 9 8 7 6 5 4 3 2
Printed in the United States of America

God Is a
Good God

God is not the author of sickness and disease. He is good, and He desires good things for His children!

The Bible tells us that "the thief's purpose is to steal and kill and destroy," but Jesus has come to give us "life in all its fullness" (John 10:10). It is the devil who would like to pull a "sneak attack" on God's people by bringing the high risk of disease—as well as the fear and worry associated with elevated cholesterol levels.

But God has provided ways to prevent this attack through the wonderful resources He has provided in His natural creation. If you have received a diagnosis of high cholesterol and all of the warnings, risks and fear that such a report brings, this Bible Cure book is for you!

Good vs. Bad

The Bible says in James 1:17 that "whatever is good and perfect comes to us from God above." Interestingly, as I will point out later in this book, there is such a thing as "good" cholesterol as well as "bad" cholesterol.

The good cholesterol we have in our bodies protects us from heart disease, helps remove the "bad" cholesterol and is God's design for our bodies. But elevating the "bad" cholesterol— which causes arterial blockage, heart attacks and strokes—is usually due to our wrong choices of foods. However, it can be lowered, especially by caring for our bodies through diet, exercise and natural supplements, which God has provided in the natural world.

A Natural and Spiritual Cure

Almost all cases of high cholesterol can be dealt with through therapeutic lifestyle changes such as diet, physical activity and weight loss. In fact, I would recommend that you follow these changes for twelve weeks before even considering the use of medication! Always make any therapeutic lifestyle changes under the care of your own physician.

In other words, God has already provided what you need, but you must take the first step toward a new, healthy lifestyle. Medication may not be necessary, but trusting in God and following His directives always are. This Bible Cure book will provide you with hope and encouragement as well as practical solutions to help you begin to lower your cholesterol and walk in the divine health that God has planned for you.

First Corinthians 6:19 tells us that our bodies are the temples of the Holy Spirit; therefore, we should treat them with the reverence that a dwelling place for God's presence deserves. Taking care of your body by eating right and following an exercise plan is important to lowering your cholesterol levels. Also in this book, you will

uncover God's divine plan of health
for body, soul and spirit
through modern medicine, good nutrition
and the medicinal power
of Scripture and prayer.

From this Bible Cure book you will gain an understanding of what your cholesterol levels mean, as well as discover God's strategic plan for keeping your "good" levels high and your "bad" levels low as you read the following chapters:

You don't have to accept a "bad report" from the doctor as a life sentence! With God's help and the knowledge of His natural remedies, you can lower your cholesterol levels and live out all the days God has planned for you—in complete health and vigor.

It is my prayer that these powerful godly insights will bring health, wholeness and spiritual refreshing to you. May they deepen your fellowship with God and strengthen your ability to worship and serve Him.

—Don Colbert, M.D.

A Bible Cure Prayer
FOR YOU

Heavenly Father, open my eyes to see the ways You have provided for me to lower my cholesterol naturally. Give me discernment to know which supplements I should take. Thank You for Your peace that frees me from anxiety and worry as I trust You for my healing from high cholesterol. In Jesus' name, amen.

Chapter 1

Knowledge Is Power!

The Bible tells us that God forgives all of our sins and heals all of our diseases (Ps. 103:3). Many diseases from which He longs to set us free have their roots in high levels of LDL (or "bad") cholesterol in the body. Coronary heart disease is most often associated with this problem, but other health problems, such as peripheral vascular disease and strokes, are related to high cholesterol as well.

Coronary heart disease accounts for approximately 500,000 deaths per year, and an estimated 102.3 million American adults have cholesterol levels above 200, which is above a healthy level. Of this number, 41.3 million have levels of 240 and higher, which puts them at high risk for heart disease.[1]

The reason that high cholesterol is so insidious

is that it is a "silent killer." Many people have no idea that their cholesterol levels are elevated until they have them checked. There may be no outward sign in your body that you have high cholesterol, though you may be walking around with a "ticking time bomb" inside just waiting to go off. Prolonged elevated levels of cholesterol may eventually lead to plaque in the coronary arteries, which can block blood flow to the heart, causing a heart attack, or hamper blood flow to the brain, causing a stroke.

Hosea 4:6 declares, "My people are destroyed for lack of knowledge" (KJV). With heart disease being the number-one killer in the United States, and high cholesterol being one of the primary causes of coronary disease,[2] it is extremely important to have your cholesterol levels checked regularly, at least every five years after age twenty. Don't let ignorance open the door to heart disease! Just because you can't feel it doesn't mean that it might not be there.

> *Praise the LORD, I tell myself, and never forget the good things he does for me. He forgives all my sins and heals all my diseases.*
> —PSALM 103:2–3

Gaining physical and spiritual refreshing and renewal requires careful wisdom from God.

Godly wisdom is a vital key to restoration for your body, as Scripture affirms: "But the excellency of knowledge is, that wisdom giveth life to them that have it" (Eccles. 7:12, KJV).

A key reason for writing this Bible Cure book is to provide you with the wisdom you need to enjoy the health and strength of total renewal. Begin by building a foundation of knowledge from which to gain dynamic wisdom to renew your health.

Even if you are a young person, you should still schedule regular appointments with your doctor—especially to check your cholesterol levels. We are discovering that atherosclerosis, the buildup of plaque in the arteries, actually begins in childhood. In fact, autopsies of American soldiers in their late teens and early twenties who were killed in the Korean War revealed advanced development of atherosclerosis.[3]

Fortunately, I have found that high cholesterol levels are usually easily managed with diet, nutrition and lifestyle changes. Only in rare cases have I seen the need for intervention through medication.

Maintaining a Healthy Lifestyle

I believe that the epidemic of high cholesterol levels in the United States today is due primarily to our poor nutritional choices. America's obsession with fast foods—including cheeseburgers, fried chicken, tacos, french fries and pizza—has led to widespread obesity and health problems, and our passion for sugar and saturated fats has continued to grow in spite of these health problems.

In 1970, Americans spent approximately $6 billion on fast food. In the year 2000, that figure skyrocketed to over $110 billion. In fact, more money is spent on fast food by Americans than on personal computers, computer software, new cars, higher education, newspapers, magazines, movies, books, videos and recorded music *combined.*[4]

> *He personally carried away our sins in his own body on the cross so we can be dead to sin and live for what is right. You have been healed by his wounds!*
> —1 PETER 2:24

The McDonald's Corporation actually spends more money on marketing and advertising than any other brand in the world—even replacing Coca-Cola as the world's most recognizable brand name. A survey of American schoolchildren revealed that 96 percent were able to identify Ronald McDonald—only Santa Claus had a higher degree of recognition![5]

Today's typical American consumes about three hamburgers and four orders of french fries every week. Even when we do decide to "eat healthy" by purchasing food from the grocery store, the benefits aren't much better: The majority of the processed, canned and packaged foods in our supermarkets are loaded with saturated, hydrogenated and partially hydrogenated fats, salt, sugar, highly processed carbohydrates and calories.

Why do we continue to buy more and more of the very items that are slowly killing us? The answer may surprise you. Processed and packaged food companies hire some of the brightest minds to study consumer psychology and demographics. And they employ brilliant chemists to ensure that you won't be satisfied with just a small amount of their product. In other words, they make sure that "you can't eat just one." Fast foods and processed foods are marketed on TV, in magazines and on billboards so that they are kept continually before your eyes, reinforcing unhealthy addictions to these foods.

Many years ago, some of the tobacco companies changed the chemical makeup of their products in order to build their business by increasing consumption. And by enticing children to smoke, they were able to create lifelong customers. Though they have not been allowed to continue this practice, it is interesting to note that tobacco companies have now begun to purchase the major brands of addictive processed foods. For example, in 2001, Phillip Morris, the world's largest tobacco company, purchased several of the most popular food brands—including Oreo cookies, Ritz crackers and Lifesavers candy—making it the world's second largest food company, just after Nestle's, Inc.[6]

The food industry has spent millions of dollars on the research of "fat-free fats." This costly practice reflects the desire of Americans to "want their cake and eat the whole thing too"—quite literally. We want something that looks like fat, tastes and feels like fat, has the creamy texture of fat—but doesn't have the calories of fat. Approximately 87 percent of

> *Pay attention, my child, to what I say. Listen carefully. Don't lose sight of my words. Let them penetrate deep within your heart, for they bring life and radiant health to anyone who discovers their meaning.*
> —PROVERBS 4:20–22

American adults eat either reduced-fat, low-fat or sugar-free food products. Sadly, many continue to gain weight, and their cholesterol levels continue to rise.[7]

Are You at Risk?

At first, all of this may sound like bad news. But it cannot be all bad if it inspires you to have your cholesterol levels checked regularly!

In May 2001, the National Cholesterol Education Program released its new set of guidelines regarding cholesterol levels. Unfortunately, their report shows that since 1993, the number of patients with abnormal cholesterol levels has tripled. They recommend a complete lipoprotein profile, or "lipid panel," for all Americans who are twenty years of age or older, to be done at least every five years. This lipid panel consists of the following screening tests:

1. Total cholesterol level
2. LDL cholesterol level
3. HDL cholesterol level
4. Triglyceride level[8]

The following numbers are the standard cholesterol measures, given in milligrams per deciliter. If your number is at the borderline level, you should take immediate steps to change your diet and lifestyle. If you have reached the high or very high level, you are at an increasingly elevated risk for serious health problems. You should follow the advice in this book and seek attention from your physician.

LDL CHOLESTEROL
   Desirable: Less than 100
   Near optimal: 100–129
   Borderline high: 130–159
   High: 160–189
   Very high: 190 or above

HDL CHOLESTEROL
   Desirable: 40 or above

TOTAL CHOLESTEROL
   Desirable: 200 or below
   Borderline: 200–239
   High: 240 or above

TRIGLYCERIDES
   Desirable: 150 or below
   Borderline: 150–199
   High: 200–499
   Very high: 500 or above

Risk Factors

If you have any form of arterial disease such as coronary artery disease, an abdominal aortic aneurysm, any arterial disease or calf pain due to poor circulation, the LDL cholesterol goal should be to maintain less than 100 mg/dl.

If you have two or more of the following risk factors, your LDL cholesterol goal should be less than 130 mg/dl. These risk factors include:

1. Age in men of forty-five or older; age in women of fifty-five or older
2. Low HDL cholesterol levels of 40 mg/dl or below
3. A history of cigarette smoking
4. Hypertension, a blood pressure reading greater than 140/90 or the need for antihypertensive medication
5. A family history of premature coronary disease—heart disease that occurs in a male relative fifty-five years old or younger or a female relative sixty-five years old or younger

If you have *any* of these risk factors, you should make some lifestyle changes, including diet, exercise and weight loss. I personally

recommend that my patients lower LDL cholesterol to 100 mg/dl or lower by following the
recommendations in this book.

Knowledge Is Power!

The fact that God's people are destroyed by lack of
knowledge is never more apparent than in the case
of high cholesterol. But God has given us the tools
we need to combat this silent killer. Knowledge,
wisdom and discipline are all important:

- *Knowledge* to understand the necessary
  dietary changes
- *Wisdom* to make the right choices
- *Discipline* to follow through

Our bodies are the temples of the Holy Spirit (1
Cor. 3:16). Let's not "trash" them by consuming
fast foods, junk foods and excessive amounts of
sugar and fat. The Bible says that we will reap what
we sow (Gal. 6:7–8). Many of us "sow" the bad
seeds of overeating and lack of exercise, and we
reap a harvest of high cholesterol, obesity, hypertension, Type 2 diabetes and heart disease. Have
your cholesterol checked by your physician, and
then begin to maintain a healthy lifestyle, planting
good seeds so that you may reap a harvest of divine
health and a long and vital life!

A BIBLE CURE PRAYER
FOR YOU

Dear Lord Jesus Christ, I thank You that You have provided the knowledge that I need to walk in the divine health that You desire for me to have. I will not allow the devil to gain a foothold in my life through the "sneak attack" of high cholesterol. Instead, I ask You to provide me with the knowledge of what will bring health to my body, the wisdom to make the right choices and the discipline and self-control to carry out those choices. In Jesus' mighty name I pray, amen.

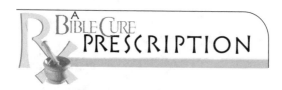

What Are Your Risk Factors?

Check the boxes for the risk factors you have, and then add up your total:

- ❏ If you are a man, are you over the age of forty-five? If you are a woman, are you over the age of fifty-five?

- ❏ Do you have HDL cholesterol levels of 40 mg/dl or below?

- ❏ Do you have a history of cigarette smoking?

- ❏ Do you have hypertension, a blood pressure reading of greater than 140/90 or the need for antihypertensive medication?

- ❏ Do you have a family history of premature coronary disease?

If you have two or more of these risk factors, and if your cholesterol level is elevated, make a commitment to follow the recommendations in this book to lower your cholesterol.

Chapter 2

The Jekyll-and-Hyde Nutrient of the Body

I f you recall the story of Dr. Jekyll and Mr. Hyde, you know that they were one and the same person—only with two very different personalities. One was a relatively kind doctor, but the other was an evil monster who emerged in certain situations. In much the same way, cholesterol can be considered the Jekyll-and-Hyde nutrient of your body. There is a good type of cholesterol (HDL)—which can lower your blood pressure and prevent disease—and there is a bad type of cholesterol (LDL) that is very detrimental to your health.

What Is Cholesterol?

Cholesterol itself is actually a soft, waxy, white substance that is found in animal food products such as red meat, poultry, eggs and dairy products. We need cholesterol to help create cell membranes for the approximately 60 to 100 trillion cells in our bodies. Cholesterol is also essential for the formation of steroid hormones, such as testosterone, progesterone and estrogen. It is necessary for the formation of bile acids and in the conversion of sunlight to vitamin D for your body's use.

About 1,000 mg of cholesterol are produced by the liver each day—all that the human body really needs to function. But Americans consume approximately another 400 to 500 mg each day in their diets.

> *But he was wounded and crushed for our sins. He was beaten that we might have peace. He was whipped, and we were healed!*
> —ISAIAH 53:5

Because cholesterol is soluble only in fat and cannot be dissolved in the bloodstream, it requires special carriers to transport it in the blood. These carriers are proteins, which encapsulate the cholesterol or *lipo;* thus they are called *lipoproteins.* It is through the presence of these lipoproteins that we can determine a person's cholesterol levels.

Let's look at several of these lipoproteins and see how they affect the cholesterol levels in your body.

HDL cholesterol (a.k.a. "Dr. Jekyll")

HDL (high-density lipoprotein) is responsible for transporting one-third to one-fourth of the cholesterol—away from the arteries and back to the liver where it is eliminated from the body. HDL actually removes cholesterol from the arterial lining, which can build up in the arteries, forming plaque, and cause coronary disease and heart attacks. For this reason, HDL cholesterol is referred to as the good, "Dr. Jekyll" side of cholesterol.

As I mentioned, HDL acts like a police officer patrolling our arteries, carrying cholesterol out of the arteries and depositing it in the liver so that it can be removed from the body. The higher the level of HDL, the lower the risk of heart disease.

It is well known that regular aerobic exercise, small amounts of red wine (one to two 4-ounce glasses a day) and the B vitamin niacin all raise HDL levels. New research is showing that dark chocolate is able to raise HDL cholesterol also. One ounce of dark chocolate contains 10 times more antioxidants than a strawberry, according to Penny Kris Etherton, N.D., Ph.D., professor of nutrition at Penn State University.

LDL cholesterol (a.k.a. "Mr. Hyde")

LDL (low-density lipoprotein) is the primary

carrier of cholesterol in the blood. If too much LDL is circulating, it can slowly build up as plaque in the arteries and can be especially dangerous in those arteries that supply blood to the heart and the brain. Clogged arteries in these areas can lead to deadly heart attacks and strokes. You will soon learn what raises LDL cholesterol and how to lower it.

What's My Cholesterol Ratio?

Your doctor will determine your cholesterol ratio by dividing your total cholesterol level by your HDL number. This gives him an idea of what your risk for coronary disease due to cholesterol actually is. The ideal ratio to reach is 3.5 to 1 or lower. Decreasing just one unit from this ratio can dramatically reduce your risk for a heart attack.

Other Important Risk Factors

Several other risk factors for heart disease should be checked by your physician—these are not included in a standard lipid panel.

Homocysteine levels

Homocysteine is an amino acid that, when elevated, is a potent oxidant of LDL (bad) cholesterol. While everyone has homocysteine in his or her blood, genetic inheritance is the most common reason for elevated homocysteine levels. Vitamin B_{12} and folic acid help to convert homocysteine to the essential amino acid methionine. And Vitamin B_6 helps to break down homocysteine to a harmless by-product. Because of the potential for injury to the lining of blood vessels when homocysteine levels are elevated, I recommend that you take a supplement like Divine Health Healthy Heart Formula to lower homocysteine levels. (See Appendix B for more information.)

Ultrasensitive or high-sensitive C-reactive protein levels

This particular protein is produced when chronic inflammation is present. It is a good predictor of cardiovascular disease because it often points to inflammation in the coronary arteries. Coronary artery disease is also a chronic inflammatory process in the arterial wall, similar to arthritis, which is a chronic inflammation of joints. Bacteria such as *Chlamydia pneumoniae, CMV, H. pylori, Borrelia burgdorferi* (Lyme disease) and so forth may be the cause of smoldering infection in the coronary arteries, indicated by the elevated ultrasensitive C-reactive protein.

Fibrinogen levels

Fibrinogen is a protein in the blood that is necessary for blood clotting to take place. Elevated fibrinogen levels increase the risk of coronary artery disease about two to three times. When fibrinogen adheres to the arterial wall, it signals platelets to clump together, which can eventually cause a buildup of soft plaque or a clot. Fibrinogen levels tend to increase with increased body weight, advancing age, high blood pressure, increased stress and smoking. If your fibrinogen level is over 300, you have a much higher risk of developing heart disease.

Lipoprotein (a)

Lipoprotein (a) is an especially dangerous lipoprotein, but surprisingly, few doctors check this cholesterol level in their patients' blood. High levels of lipoprotein (a) have been shown to dramatically increase the risk of heart disease. In fact, one study at Oxford University discovered that subjects with the highest levels of lipoprotein (a) had a 70 percent greater risk of having a heart attack within the next ten years![1]

It is critically important that you ask your doctor to check the levels of lipoprotein (a) in your bloodstream. The next time you have your cholesterol checked, ask your physician if this test is included, and if not, request it. Remember the words of Hosea: "My people are destroyed for lack of knowledge" (Hos. 4:6, KJV). Know what is going on in your body, and don't let the devil gain a foothold in your life through a lack of information about your health!

Triglycerides

Elevated triglyceride levels are linked with an increased risk of coronary disease and heart attack. These levels should also be checked by your doctor the next time he performs a routine lipid panel.

A BIBLE CURE HEALTH TIP

AmScot Medical Labs, Inc. in Cincinnati, Ohio, is able to perform all of these tests, including a lipid panel, for a very reasonable fee. Your physician can order the Comprehensive Cardiovascular Risk Assessment by calling 800-851-1708.

The Danger of Oxidation

Have you ever wondered why an apple turns brown or a nail rusts when left out in the weather too long? The answer is *oxidation.* When something is oxidized, it is combined with oxygen or gives up hydrogen or electrons. When bad cholesterol or LDL cholesterol loses electrons to oxygen, it also becomes oxidized.

Polyunsaturated fats oxidize much faster than monounsaturated fats. That is why these fats become rancid so quickly. When polyunsaturated oils such as corn oil, safflower oil, sunflower oil and others are used in cooking, and especially deep frying, oxidation occurs even faster. Oxidation also occurs in your arteries as free radicals attack the polyunsaturated fats, which are carried in LDL cholesterol.

Oxidized cholesterol is much more likely to form plaque in an artery or on arterial walls. As fats are broken down through oxidation, they form substances that promote blood clotting and cause inflammation—all of which make blood flow more difficult.

> *O Lord, you alone can heal me; you alone can save. My praises are for you alone!*
> —Jeremiah 17:14

Eating antioxidant foods such as berries, red grapes, vegetables and so forth and taking antioxidant vitamins are extremely important in preventing oxidation and reducing the risk of heart disease. In the rest of this book, we will look at foods you *should eat* to promote healthy cholesterol levels as well as foods you *should avoid* to help reduce your bad cholesterol levels. Finally, we will consider supplemental strategies that can help your body be restored to health and block the enemy's "sneak attack."

Remember what God has said in His Word: "Dear friend, I am praying that all is well with you and that your body is as healthy as I know your soul is" (3 John 2). God wants you to walk in health—and that includes healthy cholesterol levels.

A BIBLE CURE PRAYER
FOR YOU

Dear Lord Jesus, thank You for Your love and for Your healing power. Thank You that above all things You desire both my soul and my body to prosper and to be in health.

Thank You for the doctors and the knowledge they will gain to help me through the cholesterol screening tests they perform. Lord, help us to use this knowledge to take the necessary steps to keep my cholesterol levels in a healthy range.

Lord, I give my life and my body to You. I am Yours, and I know that You have good things planned for me. In Jesus' name I pray, amen.

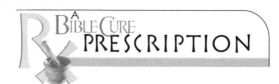

Record the cholesterol levels from your last doctor visit.

HDL _____

LDL _____

Total cholesterol _____

Triglycerides _____

What is your current cholesterol ratio?

_____ to _____

If you plan to follow the directives outlined in this book, have your levels checked again in about three months. Record your results below, and compare with previous levels:

HDL _____

LDL _____

Total cholesterol _____

Triglycerides _____

What is your cholesterol ratio at this time?

_____ to _____

Chapter 3

Foods to Avoid

Before we consider the wonderful variety of foods you should eat, let's take inventory of the foods you should avoid to maintain or restore healthy cholesterol levels. A healthy lifestyle is important for anyone to follow, but it is especially crucial for someone whose cholesterol levels register at the "borderline" or "high" range. The good news is that even if you are in this range, a few lifestyle changes can completely turn your situation around.

Even the National Cholesterol Education Program (NCEP) recommends twelve weeks of therapeutic lifestyle changes—such as diet, exercise and weight loss—before turning to medication.[1]

The NCEP recommends replacing saturated fats (such as cheese, dairy products and red meat) with monounsaturated fats (such as olive oil) and polyunsaturated fats (such as walnuts and peanuts). But to lower your cholesterol levels, you must also limit your intake of foods that elevate cholesterol.

Saturated Fats

Most Americans take in about 37 percent of their total calories from fat, which has actually decreased from 42 percent several decades ago. Even still, the American Heart Association recommends that no more than 30 percent of caloric intake should come from fats. The NCEP recommends a total fat intake of only 25 to 35 percent, with monounsaturated fats making up 20 percent of a person's total caloric intake.[2] Since polyunsaturated fats are associated with the increased oxidation of LDL cholesterol, it is wise to keep the intake of polyunsaturated fats to less than 10 percent of your total caloric intake, and saturated fats to less than 7 percent.

> *"Lord," the man said, "if you want to, you can make me well again." Jesus touched him. "I want to," he said. "Be healed!" And instantly the leprosy disappeared.*
> —MATTHEW 8:2–3

Where are the saturated fats?

Saturated fats rarely can be found in fruits and vegetables; they are primarily found in animal products. Foods high in saturated fats include most selections found at a fast-food restaurant (such as hamburgers, fried chicken strips, fried fish fillets and so forth). Dairy products such as cheese, yogurt, whole milk, ice cream, butter and cream, as well as most commercial fried foods and processed foods such as cookies, cakes, pies, pastries, doughnuts, crackers and chocolate, are typically high in saturated fats.

Saturated fats are also found in cured meat such as bacon, sausage, ham, hot dogs, cold cuts, bologna, salami and pepperoni. Duck and goose meat are also usually quite high in saturated fats. Some vegetable oils, such as coconut oil, palm kernel oil and palm oil, are also high in saturated fats.

> *Dear friend, I am praying that all is well with you and that your body is as healthy as I know your soul is.*
> —3 JOHN 2

Better choices

Making the right choices is critically important in decreasing your intake of saturated fats.

Instead of choosing to eat fast foods, fried foods, high-fat dairy foods or processed foods such as cookies, cakes, pies or other pastries, choose the low-fat alternative. For example, instead of drinking whole milk, choose skim milk; use skim-milk yogurt or cheese.

When deciding on meat, choose chicken (especially white meat) or turkey with the skin removed, fish or very lean cuts of red meat with all of its visible fat trimmed off. Bake, grill or broil your meat rather than frying it—especially avoid using a deep fryer. Instead of cold cuts, such as bologna, salami, pepperoni or even hot dogs, choose some of the leaner meats listed above. When cooking, avoid such vegetable oils as coconut oil, palm kernel oil or palm oil. Use extra-virgin olive oil or macadamia nut oil instead.

By following these simple steps and making the right choices, you'll be well on your way to decreasing saturated fats in your diet and lowering your cholesterol levels.

Hydrogenated Fats

In the 1930s a process called *hydrogenation* was developed to make liquid oils more solid. Adding hydrogen atoms to liquid fats and oils—the process called hydrogenation—made these oils stay in solid form at room temperature. They were then much less likely to become rancid, and their shelf life was greatly prolonged.

Hydrogenation changes liquid vegetable oils into a solid or spreadable fat like the margarine you spread onto a piece of toast. This process, however, alters the chemical structure of the fat to an unnatural "trans fatty acid," which becomes an enemy of the heart by raising LDL (bad) cholesterol levels and lowering the HDL (good)

> *One day while Jesus was teaching, some Pharisees and teachers of religious law were sitting nearby. . . . And the Lord's healing power was strongly with Jesus.*
> —LUKE 5:17

cholesterol levels. Trans fatty acids are also highly prone to oxidation, which causes the hardening of LDL cholesterol in the arterial wall.

Hydrogenated fats are present in margarines, shortenings and most commercial peanut butters. Margarine in stick form usually has more than 20 percent trans fatty acids, whereas most tub margarines or soft margarines only contain about 15 percent.

Smart Balance is a type of margarine with no

trans fatty acids or hydrogenated fats. It is a much better choice of margarine; however, it does contain three vegetable oils. These oils are canola oil, soybean oil and palm oil, which are not the healthiest fats.

But commercial shortenings are where the greatest problem lies—usually averaging more than 30 percent trans fatty acids. Commercial shortenings (hydrogenated and partially hydrogenated fats) are used in hundreds of processed foods, including cakes and their icing, pies, cookies, pastries, baked goods, breads, crackers, candy, nondairy creamers and many fried foods.

> *Have compassion on me, LORD, for I am weak.*
> —PSALM 6:2

Processed food companies love trans fatty acids since they provide foods with longer shelf lives and add a rich creamy texture, creating the "you-can't-eat-just-one" syndrome. Remember, the more solid the hydrogenated fat, such as stick margarine, the higher the percent of trans fatty acids it contains. Hydrogenated and partially hydrogenated fats are unnatural.

Do all that you can to remove this deadly substance from your diet by avoiding foods containing hydrogenated and partially hydrogenated fats! Read food labels carefully, and make the healthy choices to keep your cholesterol levels low.

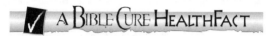

High-Cholesterol Foods

The American Heart Association has placed the daily intake limit on cholesterol at 300 mg per day. It is important to stick to this guideline; therefore, you must be on guard against foods that are high in cholesterol.

Eggs

The yolk of an average egg contains 213 mg of cholesterol—very near the daily intake limit. The American Heart Association recommends that adults only eat up to four eggs per week, but individuals with high cholesterol should limit their intake to one egg per week. There is good news, however—not everyone's cholesterol is raised by eating eggs, and some people are able to eat three eggs a day and still have normal or low cholesterol levels.

Nevertheless, if you have high cholesterol, use only egg whites or egg substitutes, such as Egg Beaters, which do not contain the yolk.

Omega-3 enriched eggs, which contain beneficial fats that help prevent heart disease, are a healthier alternative. The hens that lay these eggs are fed flaxseed meal, marine algae or fish meal instead of their regular chicken feed. However, even these eggs contain cholesterol, so you should still follow the recommendations of the American Heart Association.

Organ meats

Other foods that should be eaten in conservative amounts are all organ meats, which are very high in cholesterol. Brains, livers, kidneys, gizzards, giblets and sweetbreads from animals, chicken and fish should be avoided.

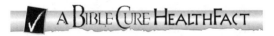

A BIBLE CURE HEALTHFACT

Four ounces of beef liver have over 500 mg of cholesterol, and 4 ounces of beef brain have about 2,000 mg of cholesterol!

Fried Foods

French fries, fish sticks, fried chicken, country fried steak, hush puppies, doughnuts, potato chips and many other foods are fried or deep-fried using saturated fats, polyunsaturated fats, hydrogenated fats or partially hydrogenated fats. Just as a sponge placed in a bucket will soak up the water, chicken, french fries, onion rings and other foods placed in buckets of grease soak it up. This dramatically multiplies our fat consumption. While there are dangers in eating saturated, hydrogenated and partially hydrogenated fats, frying foods in polyunsaturated fats is even more dangerous because it causes greater oxidation of the LDL cholesterol. If you cannot avoid frying your food, choose to stir-fry it over a low heat using olive oil, macadamia nut oil or a small amount of butter.

Carbohydrates

Carbohydrates are the most widely consumed nutrient in the world. Unfortunately Americans consume way too many highly *processed* carbohydrates, which in turn elevates insulin levels in the body. The body responds to elevated insulin levels by overproducing cholesterol, thus contributing to the high-cholesterol problem.

It's easy to lower excess insulin in your body. Simply limit or avoid highly processed and refined carbohydrates and simple sugars. By doing so, you can decrease LDL cholesterol production in your liver.

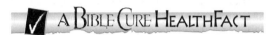

A BIBLE CURE HEALTHFACT

The top twenty sources of carbohydrates in the American diet include:

1. Potatoes, mashed or baked
2. White bread
3. Cold breakfast cereal
4. Dark bread
5. Orange juice
6. Bananas
7. White rice
8. Pizza
9. Pasta
10. Muffins
11. Fruit punch
12. Sodas
13. Apples
14. Skim milk
15. Pancakes
16. Table sugar
17. Jam
18. Cranberry juice
19. French fries
20. Candy[3]

HEALTHFACT HEALTHFACT HEALTHFACT HEALTHFACT HEALTHFACT HEALTHFACT HEALTHFACT

Glycemic Index

The glycemic index ranks foods on a scale from 0 to 100 according to whether or not they will raise blood sugar levels dramatically, moderately or just slightly. That means it measures how quickly different carbohydrates enter into the bloodstream. The faster they enter, the greater the effect on raising insulin secretion, which in turn increases cholesterol production.

Glucose (sugar) produces the greatest rise in blood sugar levels. Therefore its glycemic index is 100. Low glycemic foods have a glycemic index less than 55. (See Appendix A for the glycemic index of common foods.)

The glycemic index of most carbohydrates is influenced mainly by three factors:

1. *Soluble fiber:* The more soluble fiber a carbohydrate contains, the lower the glycemic index.
2. *Fat:* The more fat (good fats are recommended) eaten with a carbohydrate, the lower the glycemic index.
3. *Glucose:* The more glucose a carbohydrate contains, the higher the glycemic index.

A good rule of thumb is that most highly refined, man-made carbohydrates have high glycemic indexes, and foods that are in their natural state generally have lower ones. It is very important to avoid eating too many foods with a high glycemic index to maintain or restore normal cholesterol levels.

Insulin levels can also be elevated by consuming stimulants such as caffeine (coffee, tea or sodas), chocolate and even diet products. Stress also contributes to elevated insulin levels.

A kind of domino effect happens: Stimulants, as well as stress, all cause the adrenal glands to release adrenaline and cortisol. These hormones then trigger the release of the body's sugar stores into the bloodstream. The body then senses the need for more insulin to be released to lower sugar levels. The elevated insulin level then triggers the body to overproduce cholesterol.

> *Jesus traveled throughout Galilee teaching in the synagogues, preaching everywhere the Good News about the Kingdom. And he healed people who had every kind of sickness and disease.*
> —MATTHEW 4:23

This is the reason many individuals are unable to control their cholesterol; they are unknowingly eating foods, drinking beverages and even taking medications that are elevating insulin levels, ultimately causing their cholesterol levels to rise, too.

A Commitment

If that sounds like you, you may need to lay some of these foods on the altar for a period of time in order to lower your cholesterol level and regain your health. But remember that every step you take to lower your cholesterol levels—however difficult—is a step toward a healthier, longer life.

> O LORD my God,
> I cried out to
> you for help, and
> you restored
> my health.
> —PSALM 30:2

That was the bad news—now comes the good news. In the next chapter we will take a look at some delicious foods you should eat to lower your cholesterol levels.

A BIBLE CURE PRAYER
FOR YOU

Lord, I come before You today, asking You to give me Your guidance and wisdom in choosing the foods I place in my body. I ask You for a spirit of self-control as I lay my fleshly desires before You on this altar. Help me to be strong in the face of temptation and to make the right choices in order to maintain a healthy temple where Your Spirit may dwell. In Jesus' name I pray, amen.

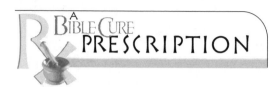

A BIBLE CURE PRESCRIPTION

Complete the following list of foods you need to avoid:

List below the saturated fats you regularly consume.

_____

_____

_____

_____

_____

List the fried foods you are willing to eliminate.

_____

_____

_____

_____

_____

_____

List refined carbohydrates you eat regularly.

_____

_____

_____

_____

_____

_____

_____

_____

_____

_____

_____

_____

_____

Ask God to help you reduce or avoid the foods on
these lists until your cholesterol levels improve.

Chapter 4

Foods You
Should Eat

As we have seen, most processed foods will dramatically raise cholesterol levels. Conversely, foods eaten in their natural state—such as fruits and vegetables—can help to *lower* cholesterol levels.

Fabulous Fiber

Foods high in soluble fiber are important to lower cholesterol levels. Two basic types of fiber exist: *soluble fiber,* which lowers cholesterol, and *insoluble fiber,* which does not. Foods high in soluble fiber include the following: beans, peas, lentils, ground flaxseed, psyllium husks and high-fiber cereals such as oat bran, rice bran and oatmeal.

Many fruits and vegetables are also high in soluble fiber, including apples, grapefruit and strawberries, and vegetables rich in pectin, including carrots, artichokes, cabbage, beans, brussels sprouts and peas. Artichokes are especially good for lowering cholesterol levels because they contain a substance called *cynarin,* which causes the liver to produce more bile. This is significant because excess cholesterol is eliminated from the body through bile.

Start Right
With a Good Breakfast!

Every morning, I grind up 1–2 tablespoons of flaxseed in a coffee grinder and add them to my protein shake. Flaxseed is a delicious source of soluble fiber. High-fiber cereals are also a great way of obtaining your soluble fiber. One excellent high-fiber cereal is Kellogg's Bran Buds with psyllium. I also recommend Kashi (Go-Lean or Good Friends) or just plain old-fashioned oatmeal. If you do not like any of these cereals, choose a cereal with at least 3 grams of fiber that is low in fat and sugar. Use skim milk, soy milk, almond milk or rice milk. Add fruit to your cereal as often as you can, such as strawberries, blueberries, sliced apples or other low-glycemic fruits that are rich in pectin.

The average American consumes only about 10–12 grams of fiber per day. We should be consuming at least 25–35 grams per day.

Many studies have shown the benefits of adding soluble fiber to the diet. One study at Stanford University School of Medicine found that individuals who consumed just 5 grams of soluble fiber per day for a month decreased their LDL cholesterol levels by 5.6 percent. Those who consumed 15 grams of soluble fiber lowered their LDL cholesterol by 14.9 percent.[1] By simply selecting foods higher in soluble fiber with each meal, you can achieve a dramatic impact.

A word of caution: Increase your intake of soluble fiber gradually, or you may experience gas and bloating. To decrease the occurrence of gas caused by legumes, I recommend you soak your beans overnight and then discard the water before cooking them.

HEALTHFACT HEALTHFACT HEALTHFACT HEALTHFACT HEALTHFACT HEALTHFACT HEALTHFACT

Olive Oil and Foods High in Monounsaturated Fats

Consuming foods that are high in monounsaturated fats is a good way to lower your cholesterol levels.

Olive oil is composed primarily of monounsaturated fats—specifically oleic acid, which makes up about 75 percent of the fat in olive oil. Olive oil has been shown both to help decrease LDL or bad cholesterol levels and to increase HDL or good cholesterol levels. Extra-virgin olive oil and virgin olive oil also help to block the oxidation of LDL cholesterol.

If you haven't already done so, begin to substitute extra-virgin olive oil in your diet for oils with polyunsaturated and saturated fats. Instead of using butter on bread, try dipping it in extra-virgin olive oil with cracked pepper and garlic. Instead of regular salad dressings, use extra-virgin olive oil and balsamic vinegar. Also, sauté foods with olive oil and add olive oil to sauces in place of butter. You will find the taste is delicious.

A BIBLE CURE HEALTH TIP

Experts have found that extra-virgin olive oil is more effective than regular olive oil in preventing the oxidation of LDL cholesterol. Whenever possible, use either extra-virgin or virgin olive oil in place of plain olive oil.

Nuts and Avocados

Almonds and macadamia nuts are also high in monounsaturated fats that help to lower cholesterol. These tasty nuts can be added sparingly to salads and fat-free yogurt or sprinkled on pancakes, cereals or waffles. One word of caution: Because almonds and macadamia nuts are high in calories, you should not eat them by the handfuls!

Another good food that contains monounsaturated fat and helps to lower LDL cholesterol is the avocado. Avocados, like olive oil, are rich in oleic acid. However, they are very high in fat also and should be limited if you are overweight or obese. Avocados, used in moderation

> *He comforts us in all our troubles so that we can comfort others. When others are troubled, we will be able to give them the same comfort God has given us.*
> —2 Corinthians 1:4

in salads or spread over a sandwich in place of mayonnaise, will add wonderful flavor while they work to lower LDL cholesterol in your body.

The Canola Oil Controversy

Canola oil is also rich in monounsaturated fats. In fact, many experts recognize canola oil as having the best fatty-acid ratio of any oil. This simply means that it has the lowest level of saturated fat (only 7 percent) and is high in monounsaturated fats (61 percent).

However, canola oil is a source of controversy among nutritionists. Dr. Mary G. Enig, Ph.D., one of the top biochemists in the country, finds that canola oil has to be partially hydrogenated or refined before it is used commercially. Consequently it becomes a source of trans fatty acids, sometimes at very high and dangerous levels.[2] Other experts agree that a large portion of canola oil used in processed food has been hardened through the hydrogenation process, causing levels of trans fatty acids as high as a whopping 40 percent!

Canola oil does actually hydrogenate better than corn or soybean oil—and this allows it a longer shelf life in processed foods as well as a crispier texture in both cookies and crackers. The trans fatty acids in canola oil are generally not listed on the label, but they are almost always present. Because an increased intake of hydrogenated fats increases LDL cholesterol as well as its oxidation, I don't recommend canola oil or processed foods that contain canola oil. Instead, purchase food products that contain extra-virgin olive oil.

Superior Soy

Studies reveal that a total daily intake of 25 grams of soy protein as part of a low-fat diet significantly lowers both total cholesterol and LDL cholesterol levels. Twenty-five grams of soy protein is equal to about 8 ounces of soy milk.[3] Soy foods help lower cholesterol and decrease the risk for heart disease, and in 1999, the FDA allowed food manufacturers of soy protein products to claim it reduces the risk of coronary heart disease.[4]

Many different types of soy protein products are available, including soy milk, soy nuts, isolated soy protein and soy flour. Meats made with soy include burgers, sausage, bacon and frankfurters. Other soy products include soy cheese, soy yogurt, tempeh and tofu. If you have high cholesterol, you can begin to substitute soy protein for animal protein in your diet, which will cause a significant reduction in your LDL cholesterol levels.

> *The leaves of the tree were for the healing of the nations.*
> —Revelation 22:2, KJV

Remarkable Red Wine

No other food or beverage can decrease your overall risk of a heart attack more than wine, primarily because it contains *resveratrol.* Resveratrol is a substance found in grapes that helps prevent fungus from growing on the grapes' skin. In the human body, resveratrol has been proven to increase HDL cholesterol, and it also inhibits the oxidation of LDL cholesterol.

Red wine is much more powerful than white wine for raising HDL (good) cholesterol. It contains fifty to one hundred times more resveratrol than white wine does. In addition, red wine has more than one hundred different flavonoids with antioxidant and anti-inflammatory properties.

However, red wine must be consumed in moderate amounts. The U.S. Department of Agriculture defines "moderation in alcohol intake" as no more than one 4-ounce glass per day for women and no more than two of the same size per day for men.[5] However, certain individuals—including pregnant women or those with liver disease, congestive heart failure or active ulcer disease—should avoid alcohol completely. Those with substance abuse problems should also abstain. Finally, no one should drink alcohol—not even wine—and drive.

If you have elevated cholesterol levels, consult your physician to see if red wine in moderation is right for you. For individuals who do not drink alcohol, red wine is available in supplement form, such as red wine capsules or a supplement called *French Paradox*. These capsules contain no alcohol but do contain many of the beneficial properties of red wine. Other alternatives include nonalcoholic red wine and grape juice, but I do not usually recommend them because of their high sugar levels, which could actually raise your total cholesterol.

> *The sick begged him [Jesus] to let them at least touch the fringe of his robe, and all who touched it were healed.*
> —MARK 6:56

Low-Fat Choices

You can lower your cholesterol levels dramatically without having to sacrifice enjoyable meals. Simply begin choosing lower fat alternatives.

Instead of fatty cuts of red meat, eat fish, chicken or turkey with the skin removed, or extra-lean meat with all visible fat trimmed off. Bake, grill or broil your meat instead of frying it.

And rather than buying high-fat dairy products, purchase skim milk, skim-milk cheeses and skim-milk yogurts. Better still, choose soy products as they have the added benefit of lowering your LDL cholesterol levels.

Syndrome X

As many as 22 percent of American adults—some 47 million people—may have a sinister-sounding disorder called *Syndrome X,* or "metabolic syndrome."[6] It is marked by abdominal obesity; a high triglyceride level (greater than 150 mg/dl); a low HDL good cholesterol level (less than 40 mg/dl in men and less than 50 mg/dl in women); a blood pressure reading of greater than or equal to 130/85 and a fasting sugar level greater than or equal to 110 mg/dl.

Since high levels of triglycerides combined with low HDL levels are associated with an increased risk of heart disease, a person with Syndrome X could be headed for trouble.

If you have this condition, you should stop all consumption of alcoholic beverages in addition to any of the sugars and refined carbohydrates. Begin a weight-loss program immediately, especially to lose the abdominal fat, sometimes referred to as the "apple-shaped" obesity. Also start a regular aerobic exercise program, such as taking a brisk walk three to four times a week for at least twenty minutes.

If you are thirty-five years of age or older with cardiovascular risk factors, make sure that you have been medically cleared by your physician before starting any exercise program.

Get Moving!

Aerobic exercises can help lower the levels of LDL bad cholesterol in your body. These activities use the large muscle groups of the body in repetitive motion for a sustained period of time. They include brisk walking, jogging, aerobic dancing, cycling, swimming, skating, gliding machine, stair stepping, rowing and cross-country skiing. They may also include a game of tennis, basketball, racquetball or any other vigorous sport.

A BIBLE CURE HEALTH TIP

On its own, regular aerobic exercise lowers the risk of coronary heart disease and helps to decrease body weight, lower blood pressure, lower blood triglyceride levels, lower LDL (bad) cholesterol levels and raise HDL (good) cholesterol levels.

You can lower your LDL cholesterol levels much more by combining these exercises with a diet that is:

- Low in saturated and hydrogenated fats

- Low in cholesterol, sugar and refined carbohydrates

- High in monounsaturated fats and soluble fiber

The key to success is to find an exercise that you enjoy and will do regularly. If necessary, make a commitment to exercise with a friend, and keep that exercise appointment just as you would keep any other important appointment.

It isn't difficult to lower your LDL cholesterol levels and raise your HDL levels. By choosing the right foods to eat and avoiding the wrong ones, along with adding regular exercise to your life-style, you can be on your way to a happier, healthier life.

A BIBLE CURE PRAYER
FOR YOU

Dear heavenly Father, thank You so much for Your marvelous creation. Thank You for the delicious foods You have created that not only are pleasing to my taste but also bring health to my body. Help me to increase my knowledge of the foods that will lower my cholesterol levels and restore health to my body. And, once armed with that knowledge, help me to include those foods more and more into my diet. I thank You that as I walk in obedience to Your Word and do what is best for my body, You will reward my obedience with good health and a long life upon the earth. In Jesus' name, amen.

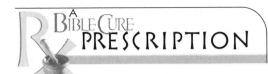

R A BIBLE CURE
PRESCRIPTION

List sources of fiber you will add to your diet.

_____

_____

_____

_____

_____

_____

_____

List sources of monounsaturated fats you will add
to your diet.

_____

_____

_____

_____

_____

_____

_____

What "new" foods listed in this chapter will you add to your diet?

_____

_____

_____

_____

_____

_____

List the exercises you will commit to doing.

_____

_____

_____

_____

How often?

_____

_____

_____

Chapter 5

Supplement Strategies for Healthy Cholesterol

As we have seen throughout this book, with God's help to implement proper diet and exercise, you can lower your cholesterol levels and live out all the days He has planned for you—in complete health and vigor. In this chapter we will consider some of the natural remedies God has placed in His creation. Formulated as supplements, when added to a healthy diet, these natural substances can restore healthy cholesterol levels to the body, often without any medical intervention.

Soluble Fiber Supplements

In the previous chapter I discussed how foods that are high in soluble fiber can greatly reduce levels of LDL cholesterol. However, many people may find it difficult to take time to prepare these kinds of foods. For these individuals, I recommend soluble-fiber supplements.

Choosing a fiber supplement

Over-the-counter fiber supplement products such as Metamucil contain psyllium husks, which are an excellent source of fiber. However, many of the liquid forms of these supplements contain sugar or NutraSweet, so be sure to read the labels. Metamucil has recently come out with a supplement in capsule form, which is an easy and convenient way to obtain your soluble fiber without unnecessarily adding sugar to your diet.

Another very good fiber supplement is *Fiber Delights,* which contains 2 grams of soluble fiber per tablet. This supplement contains inulin fiber along with fiber from the chicory root and oat bran. You should start with one tablet a day and eventually work up to one tablet three times a day with meals. This chewable fiber supplement contains neither sugar nor NutraSweet. To order, call (888) 792-0028.

Other forms of soluble fiber can be added to smoothies or mixed in cereals or oatmeal. These include oat bran, rice bran, psyllium seed, psyllium husks, guar gum and flaxseed. I grind 2 tablespoons of flaxseeds in a coffee grinder and add it to my protein smoothie each morning.

Amazing Antioxidants

As I discussed in a previous chapter, when LDL cholesterol becomes oxidized, it is much more likely to form plaque on arterial walls. For this reason, supplementation with antioxidants is extremely important to decrease any damage caused by oxidized LDL cholesterol.

Antioxidants work best when taken together as a team rather than as a single antioxidant. Several antioxidants play an extremely important role in preventing the oxidation of LDL cholesterol. One of the most important is vitamin E in its natural form (d-alpha-tocopherol), which prevents and even reverses the oxidized state of cholesterol. Other important antioxidants include lipoic acid, vitamin C, coenzyme Q_{10}, grape seed and pine bark extract and selenium.

Another way to protect against the damage of oxidation includes taking supplements of oils high in essential fatty acids. These include flaxseed oil, fish oil and evening primrose oil. These oils help to balance lipid metabolism and protect against the damage caused by oxidized cholesterol and hydrogenated fats. Be careful when purchasing these supplements, however, because many of the fish oils sold over the counter have become rancid. I recommend Divine Health Omega-3 Fatty Acids, which are nonrancid fish oils.

In addition, I also recommend that you take a comprehensive multivitamin and antioxidant formula such as Divine Health Multivitamin and Divine Health Elite Antioxidant Formula.

Divine Health Elite Antioxidant contains coenzyme Q_{10} and alpha-lipoic acid, in addition to other important antioxidants that help protect the body from the formation of damaging free radicals. Excessive free radicals are associated with aging and degenerative diseases, including heart disease and cancer. Divine Health Elite Antioxidant's specially balanced formulation will help neutralize free radicals and give you added protection. To order these products, see Appendix B at the end of this book.

Power-Packed
Policosanol

In 1964, Cuba's minister of industry created the first postrevolution, state-sponsored research center, called The Cuban Institute for Research on Sugar Cane Derivatives. Its intent was to identify sugar cane derivatives that would surpass the quality of refined white sugar. The first product identified with this potential was *policosanol.*

Policosanol is an extract of the Cuban sugar cane derived from the plant's waxy fraction. According to studies, policosanol is just as powerfully effective in lowering cholesterol, or more so, than most statin drugs, including lovastatin, simvastatin, pravastatin, gemfibrozil, Acipimox and probucol.

> *I will give you back your health and heal your wounds, says the LORD.*
> —JEREMIAH 30:17

Policosanol lowers LDL cholesterol, raises

HDL cholesterol and protects against oxidative damage to LDL cholesterol. With a dosage of just 10 mg a day—the recommended dosage—a patient's LDL cholesterol level typically will drop 20–25 percent within the first six months. And at a dosage of 20 mg a day, LDL cholesterol levels typically drop 25–30 percent, according to studies.

Because policosanol is a very safe substance to take, it can be used by the elderly, diabetic patients and even those with impaired liver functions or severe liver damage.

Note: Most policosanol supplements available in this country do not effectively lower cholesterol levels. I recommend policosanol available from Cardiovascular Research, which usually lowers cholesterol quite effectively. (See Appendix B for ordering information.)

Necessary Niacin

Niacin not only lowers total cholesterol levels, including LDL cholesterol, but it also lowers triglyceride levels and raises HDL cholesterol levels. The dose of niacin required to lower cholesterol levels is usually 1 gram taken three times a day. Or you may take a sustained-release niacin supplement such as Niaspan, at a dose of 1,000 to 3,000 mg at bedtime.

Unfortunately, because niacin may cause numerous side effects, such as flushing of the skin, ulcers, stomach irritation, elevated liver enzymes and fatigue, many people are unable to tolerate it. For these individuals, there is another form of niacin called *inositol hexaniacinate*. This form of niacin carries all the benefits of regular niacin without the side effects.

Inositol hexaniacinate has been used in Europe to lower cholesterol levels and improve blood flow in patients with intermittent calf pain due to poor circulation. Approximately 1,000 to 1,500 mg per day of inositol hexaniacinate in divided doses is usually adequate for lowering LDL cholesterol and raising HDL cholesterol levels. However, some may need a higher dose. Be sure to consult your physician first before deciding to add any natural "medications" to your lifestyle.

If you are taking medication for diabetes, monitor your blood sugar levels closely when taking any form of niacin, even inositol hexaniacinate. Divine Health Chol-Less contains inositol hexaniacinate in a 1,350-mg dosage. In addition, it contains 500 mg of gugulipid, 225 mg of guar gum and 150 mg of artichoke leaf extract. I recommend that my patients take one tablet of Divine Health Chol-Less, three times a day. (See Appendix B for ordering information.)

Fantastic Phytosterols

The National Cholesterol Education Program suggests adding hydrogenated phytosterols to your diet if initial attempts to lower cholesterol in other ways have not succeeded. Phytosterols (plant sterols) effectively interfere with small intestine absorption of cholesterol and therefore, when eaten, can lower a person's LDL cholesterol levels.

Seeds, nuts, vegetables, fruits, beans and legumes all contain adequate amounts of phytosterols that can lower your levels of LDL cholesterol. Phytosterols are also found in many products, including some margarine spreads; all vegetables and vegetable-based products contain phytosterols. Two of the newer margarine products, Benechol and Take Control, are said to lower cholesterol levels by interfering with the absorption of cholesterol from the food that is eaten with the products. Even still, Dr. Joseph Mercola has this to say about Take Control margarine: "Never forget, margarine is liquid plastic. Your brain is 50 percent fat. Do you want liquid plastic incorporated into your brain?"[1]

In their natural state, all phytosterols are bound to the fibers of the plant from which they come. And there is a better way to incorporate these phytosterols into your diet than eating a tub of margarine! As frequently as possible, try to eat foods with phytosterols as they are grown in nature, before they have been processed and refined.

Gallant Gugulipids

Gugulipids actually come from the resin of the mukul myrrh tree. The actual ingredients beneficial to the human body are the guggulsterones. Studies have demonstrated that 25 mg of guggulsterone three times a day, which is equivalent to 500 mg of a 5 percent guggulsterone extract three times a day, is effective for countering elevated cholesterol and triglyceride levels. It is believed that gugulipids work by increasing the number of hepatic LDL receptors, increasing bile secretion and decreasing cholesterol synthesis. Simply put, it helps to decrease the amount of cholesterol the body absorbs and helps to flush out the cholesterol that has been absorbed. Divine Health Chol-Less contains gugulipids. (See Appendix B for ordering information.)

Amazing Artichoke Extract

Artichokes contain cynarin, a substance that causes the liver to produce and excrete additional bile into the gallbladder and small intestine. When cynarin is combined with soluble fiber in the body, cholesterol becomes bound to the fiber and unable to be reabsorbed, and is, therefore, removed from the body with the stool. While artichokes themselves are a good source of cynarin, extracts can be made from artichokes that have a higher cynarin content. Divine Health Chol-Less contains artichoke extract. (See Appendix B for ordering information.)

Potent Pantethine

Pantethine is the active, stable form of pantothenic acid, otherwise known as vitamin B_5. It can be used to lower LDL cholesterol and triglyceride levels while increasing HDL levels. It is believed that pantethine inhibits the production of cholesterol and accelerates the breakdown of fatty acids in the body. Pantethine works best when taken at a dose of 300 mg, three times a day.

Remarkable Red Yeast Rice

Red yeast is a form of yeast that is cultivated on rice, and it contains substances very similar to the active ingredients in statin drugs, the most commonly prescribed medications for elevated cholesterol levels. Clinical trials performed on red yeast rice products showed that they were able to lower total cholesterol levels by an average of 16 percent.

Although red yeast rice is available to the public, it is not certain that these products are entirely safe. According to Dr. Andrew Weil, some red yeast rice products are contaminated with citrinin, a toxin that causes kidney damage in animals.[2] If you choose to use red yeast rice to lower your cholesterol, be sure to obtain it from a reputable nutritional supplement company, and do so *only* under the care of your physician. Be sure to have your liver checked regularly since red yeast rice can cause liver abnormalities.

Help for High Triglycerides

Fish oils, or omega-3 fats from fish, can lower triglyceride levels by as much as 30 percent.[3] In fact, fish oil is one of the most effective treatments for lowering triglyceride levels and is much safer than medical drug therapy. Fish oil contains EPA and DHA and is more beneficial than vegetable omega-3 oils such as flaxseed oil. Salmon, mackerel, sardines and herring contain more omega-3 fats than other fish, but "farm-raised" fish contain very little omega-3 oil because many farms feed their fish soybean meal.

I recommend eating three to four meals of seafood each week, consisting of the fish I listed above. But do not fry or deep-fry the fish, because that will counteract any of the benefits of the omega-3 fats.

Fish oil may also be obtained in supplement form. To lower your triglycerides, you should take approximately 3,000 mg per day of omega-3 oil. For example, if an omega-3 capsule contains 1,000 mg of fish oil, with 180 mg of it being EPA and 120 mg being DHA, then the total omega-3 oil that you are receiving from the capsule is 300 mg, and you would need to take ten capsules per day.

Another point of consideration: Most fish oil supplements sold over the counter are rancid, meaning that you will not get the beneficial effects from them that you need. A simple test to tell if a fish oil capsule is rancid is to stick a needle into it and then smell it. If it has a very "fishy" odor, it is rancid. I recommend that you use a higher grade nonrancid fish oil such as Divine Health Omega-3 Fatty Acids. It contains 720 mg of omega-3 fats per capsule. You should start with one capsule three times a day, later increasing the dosage to two capsules three times a day. (See Appendix B for ordering information.)

Medical Therapy?

Unfortunately, there are cases in which therapeutic lifestyle changes—including a proper diet, physical activity and weight loss—cannot achieve the recommended LDL cholesterol goal in a short enough period of time. After twelve weeks without a significant improvement, the National Cholesterol Education Program recommends considering the use of medication.[4]

> *Yes, your healing will come quickly. Your godliness will lead you forward, and the glory of the LORD will protect you from behind.*
> —ISAIAH 58:8

If you have followed the advice in this book and still have high cholesterol, you may have an underactive thyroid, which is called hypothyroidism. I have watched cholesterol levels as high as 400 in patients decrease to normal levels after they were placed on thyroid medication. Make sure that you have your thyroid checked if your cholesterol levels do not decrease with diet, exercise and supplementation.

The most commonly prescribed cholesterol-lowering medications are the statin drugs, which include Zocor, Mevacor, Pravachol and Lipitor. Lipitor is the best-selling drug in America, with over 57 million prescriptions for it filled in 2001. Zocor is the third best-selling drug in America. These medications work by inhibiting an enzyme that limits cholesterol synthesis, thus lowering overall cholesterol levels. While these medications can work wonders in some people, they should be avoided in those with liver disease.

Problems can arise with the statin drugs, however. Almost all of them have been associated with rare reports of *rhabdomyolysis,* a condition that results in the breakdown and release of the contents of muscle cells into the bloodstream. Symptoms of rhabdomyolysis include weakness, muscle pain, tenderness, dark urine, nausea, vomiting, fever and malaise.

Some cases of rhabdomyolysis—found in association with the use of another statin called Baycol—actually proved to be fatal. And more cases have been reported with Baycol than with any other approved statin drug. Due to these dangers, Bayer voluntarily withdrew Baycol from the U.S. market on August 8, 2001.[5]

Rhabdomyolysis can occur with any statin drug, and the risk for the condition increases when the lipid-lowering drug Lopid is combined with it.

Another side effect of statin drugs is they have been demonstrated to block the synthesis of co-enzyme Q_{10}.[6] For this reason, if you are taking a statin drug, you should also take at least 30 mg of coenzyme Q_{10} a day.

> *Don't be afraid, for I am with you. Do not be dismayed, for I am your God. I will strengthen you. I will help you. I will uphold you with my victorious right hand.*
> —ISAIAH 41:10

A Bible Cure Prayer
FOR YOU

Dear Lord, I thank You for providing natural solutions to restore my health and lower my cholesterol levels. Grant me the wisdom that I need to select the proper supplements that will serve the correct purpose in my body. Thank You for making it possible for me to walk in Your divine and perfect health. In Jesus' name, amen.

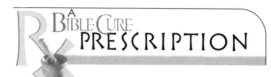

A BIBLE CURE PRESCRIPTION

It is vitally important to carefully consider which supplements are right for you to take, along with receiving your physician's counsel. List below the supplements you want to try, along with the key function of that supplement. Understanding the purpose of the supplements you take is very important. Then take your list to your physician to approve.

_____

_____

_____

_____

_____

_____

_____

_____

_____

Conclusion

It is always best if you can avoid the use of prescription medicine and use natural methods to lower your cholesterol.

Simply decrease your intake of saturated and hydrogenated fats, decrease your consumption of high-cholesterol foods and limit the amount of simple sugars and highly processed carbohydrates in your diet, and your LDL cholesterol levels will begin to decrease naturally.

Eliminate man-made, processed foods from your diet, and choose "God-made" foods such as fruits, vegetables and whole grains, which are high in soluble fiber. Begin to use extra-virgin olive oil and soy products. Choose lean meats, fish, turkey and chicken without its skin. As you prefer skim milk and skim-milk cheeses and yogurt in place of fatty cheeses, butter and whole-milk products, your cholesterol levels will come down even further.

Start a regular aerobic exercise program by walking briskly three to four times a week for twenty minutes. And take supplements such as soluble-fiber supplements, antioxidants, policosanol and Divine Health Chol-Less. (See Appendix B for ordering.) By following these simple steps, you will begin to notice a dramatic change in your cholesterol levels, and you will be on your way to a happier, healthier life!

With a little faith in a great big God, you will quickly discover that He will supply all the wisdom and resources you need—even the discipline. So get ready to enjoy greater health than you have ever had!

Appendix A

Common Foods and Their Glycemic Index[1]

Vegetables

Kidney beans	27	Corn	55
Lentils	30	New potatoes	62
Lima beans	31	French fries	75
Green peas	48	Red skinned potatoes	88
Carrots	49	Baked potato	93
Sweet potatoes	54		

Fruits

Cherries	22	Grapes	46
Grapefruit	25	Kiwi	52
Peach	30	Mango	55
Apple	38	Banana	55
Pear	38	Cantaloupe	65
Plum	39	Pineapple	66
Orange	44	Watermelon	72

Breads

Whole-grain pumpernickel 51	Croissant 67
Sour dough 52	Whole wheat 69
Stone-ground whole wheat 53	White bread 70
Pita bread 57	Bagel 72
	Rye 76

Breakfast cereals

Kellogg's Bran Buds with psyllium 45	Kellogg's All Bran with extra fiber 51
Old-fashioned oatmeal 49	Kellogg's Rice Krispies . . .82
	Kellogg's Cornflakes 84

Grains and pasta

Spaghetti 41	Rice, short grain white 72
Instant noodles 46	Crackers 81
Rice, brown 55	

Product List

Divine Health Healthy Heart Formula
Call (407) 331-7007 or visit the Web site
at www.drcolbert.com.

Policosanol from Cardiovascular Research
Call (800) 888-4585
Mention Dr. Colbert's name when calling.

Divine Health Elite Antioxidant Formula
Call (407) 331-7007 or visit the Web site
at www.drcolbert.com.

Divine Health Multivitamins
Call (407) 331-7007 or visit the Web site
at www.drcolbert.com.

Divine Health Chol-Less

Contains inositol hexaniacinate, gugulipid and
artichoke extract. Call (407) 331-7007
or visit the Web site at www.drcolbert.com.

Pantethine

Call Integrative Therapeutics at (800) 931-1709
and ask for Pantethine Plus. When prompted,
provide Dr. Colbert's code PCP-5266.

Divine Health Omega-3 Fatty Acids

Call (407) 331-7007 or visit the Web site
at www.drcolbert.com.

A PERSONAL NOTE

From Don and Mary Colbert

God desires to heal you of disease. His Word is full of promises that confirm His love for you and His desire to give you His abundant life. His desire includes more than physical health for you; He wants to make you whole in your mind and spirit as well through a personal relationship with His Son, Jesus Christ.

If you haven't met our best friend, Jesus, we would like to take this opportunity to introduce Him to you. It is very simple.

If you are ready to let Him come into your heart and become your best friend, just bow your head and sincerely pray this prayer from your heart:

> *Lord Jesus, I want to know You as my Savior and Lord. I believe You are the Son of God and that You died for my sins. I also believe You were raised from the dead and now sit at the right hand of the Father praying for me. I ask You to forgive me for my sins and change my heart so that I can*

be Your child and live with You eternally.
Thank You for Your peace. Help me to
walk with You so that I can begin to know
You as my best friend and my Lord. Amen.

If you have prayed this prayer, we rejoice with you in your decision and your new relationship with Jesus. Please contact us at pray4me@strang.com so that we can send you some materials that will help you become established in your relationship with the Lord. You have just made the most important decision of your life. We look forward to hearing from you.

Notes

Chapter 1
Knowledge Is Power!

1. The Centers for Disease Control, Preventing Heart Disease and Stroke: Addressing the Nation's Leading Killers (Atlanta, GA: CDC, 2003).
2. Ibid.
3. The Bogalusa, Louisiana, Heart Study, 1953, *Journal of the American Medical Association* 281 (February 24, 1999), 8.
4. Eric Schlosser, *Fast Food Nation* (Boston, MA: Houghton-Mifflin Company, 2001).
5. Ibid.
6. Paul Zane Pilzer, *The Wellness Revolution* (Hoboken, NJ: John Wiley & Sons, Inc., 2002).
7. Ibid.
8. National Cholesterol Education Program, Third Report of the Expert Panel, Detection, Evaluation, and Treatment of High Blood Cholesterol in Adults (Adult Treatment Panel III), 2001.

Chapter 2
The Jekyll-and-Hyde Nutrient of the Body

1. *Journal of the American Heart Association.* Journal Report 09/04/2000: "Cholesterol-Carrying Particle Tied to 70 Percent Increase in Heart Attack Risk."

Chapter 3
Foods to Avoid

1. National Cholesterol Education Program, Third Report of the Expert Panel, Detection, Evaluation, and Treatment of High Blood Cholesterol in Adults (Adult Treatment Panel III), 2001.
2. Ibid.
3. Jennie Brand-Miller, *The Glucose Revolution* (New York, NY: Marlowe and Company, 1999).

Chapter 4
Foods You Should Eat

1. C. D. Gardner, S. P. Fortmann, and R. M. Krauss, "Association of Small Low-Density Lipoprotein Particles With the Incidence of Coronary Artery Disease in Men and Women," *Journal of the American Medical Association* 276 (Sept. 18, 1996), 875.
2. M. G. Enig, *Trans Fatty Acids in the Food Supply: A Comprehensive Report Covering 60 Years of Research, 2nd Edition* (Silver Spring, MD: Enig Associates, Inc., 1995).
3. F. M. Steinberg and M. M. Braun, "Dietary Soy Isoflavones Reduce Plasma LDL Cholesterol and Atherosclerosis in a Human Apolipoprotein B Transgenic Mouse Model," *Third International Symposium on the Role of Soy in Preventing and Treating Chronic Disease,* Department of Nutrition, University of California, 1999.
4. FDA talk paper, "FDA Approves New Health Claim for

Soy Protein and Coronary Heart Disease," Food and
Drug Administration, October 20, 1999.

5. William V. Rumpler, Donna Rhodes and David J. Baer,
   "Chronic Moderate Alcohol Consumption and the
   Thermic Effect of a Meal with or without Alcohol,"
   Agricultural Research, September 26, 1995.

6. *Journal of the American Medical Association*
   (January 16, 2002).

CHAPTER 5
SUPPLEMENT STRATEGIES FOR HEALTHY CHOLESTEROL

1. Joseph Mercola, *The No-Grain Diet* (New York, NY:
   E. P. Dutton, 2003).

2. Andrew Weil, "The Cholestin Controversy," *Dr.
   Andrew Weil's Self Healing*, August 1998.

3. J. G. Coniglio, "How Does Fish Oil Lower Plasma
   Triglycerides?" *Nutr Rev* 50 (July 1992): 195–197.

4. National Cholesterol Education Program, Third
   Report of the Expert Panel, *Detection, Evaluation,
   and Treatment of High Blood Cholesterol in Adults
   (Adult Treatment Panel III)*, 2001.

5. MedWatch—Baycol Withdrawal Letter, retrieved from
   the Internet August 25, 2003, at www.fda.gov/
   medwatch/safety/2001/Baycol2.htm.

6. Bernd Wollschlaeger, "Commentary: Statin Drugs and
   Coenzyme Q_{10}," *Journal of the American Nutra-
   ceutical Association*, May 2001.

Appendix A
Common Foods and Their Glycemic Index

1. Brand-Miller, *The Glucose Revolution*.

Don Colbert, M.D., was born in Tupelo, Mississippi. He attended Oral Roberts School of Medicine in Tulsa, Oklahoma, where he received a bachelor of science degree in biology in addition to his degree in medicine. Dr. Colbert completed his internship and residency with Florida Hospital in Orlando, Florida. He is board certified in family practice and has received extensive training in nutritional medicine.

If you would like more
information about natural and
divine healing, or information about
Divine Health Nutritional Products,
you may contact
Dr. Colbert at:

DR. DON COLBERT

1908 Boothe Circle
Longwood, FL 32750
Telephone: 407-331-7007
(For ordering products only)

Dr. Colbert's Web site is
www.drcolbert.com.

Disclaimer: Dr. Colbert and the staff of Divine Health Wellness Center are prohibited from addressing a patient's medical condition by phone, facsimile or e-mail. Please refer questions related to your medical condition to your own primary care physician.

Divine Health
Chol-Less Formula

Divine Health Chol-Less Formula addresses four of the five ways an individual can maintain cholesterol levels within the normal range, the fifth being diet. Hence, with proper diet and Divine Health Chol-Less Formula, you can lower your elevated cholesterol levels. This classic formula is designed to help enhance the body's own metabolic and bile secreting mechanisms. Because these are natural ingredients, the formula will not damage the liver or reduce other vital coenzyme Q_{10} levels in the body. Three capsules contain 200 mcg of chromium, 1350 mg of inositol hexaniacinate, 500 mg of gugulipids, 225 mg of guar gum and 150 mg of artichoke extract.

Product # 112 — 90 Capsules   **$30.00**